Hair Pulling in Children:

How to Help Your Child Stop Hair Pulling

By Amy Foxwell

Table of Contents

A Word to Parents

Firstly, let me congratulate you on your pro-activeness and willingness to help your child through Trichotillomania. You have taken the first step to helping your child in their battle against hair pulling. Whether your child has been battling with Trichotillomania for many years, or has just begun to suffer from this condition, as a parent you must take an active position today in helping your child beat Trich.

I began suffering from Trich as a young child. I even remember proudly saving all of my eyelashes in a box. However, my parents did nothing at the time to deal with my condition, which eventually made it much more difficult for me in the long run. I suffered from my condition for over 35 years before finally finding a set of treatments that helped me become an 'ex-Trichster'. I can only think that if my parents had been more aware, or more supportive, I would not have suffered for so long.

Your child will need your help, encouragement, patience, guidance and wisdom. But together I know that you can beat Trich. Who knows, perhaps even your relationship will benefit from working through this difficult challenge together.

All my best for you and your child,

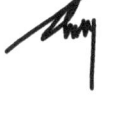

Amy Foxwell

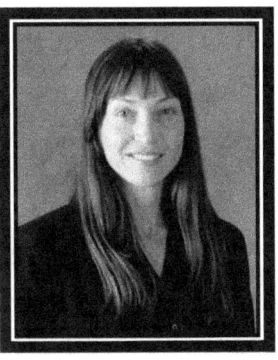

Why does my child suffer from this?

Trichotillomania is an impulse control disorder. Sufferers are unable to stop this behavior, and the behavior is often self-destructive and distressing to the sufferer.

It is important to understand from the very beginning that Trichotillomania is serious condition and more than just a nervous habit, which can be controlled through simply by deciding to stop.

Research of causes and treatments of Trichotillomania are still in the early stages, and no one is really sure what causes Trich. Most likely there are several different causes that may act separately or as a combined cause. It could be a neurobiological disorder and may be linked to one's genetic makeup. At times it is triggered by stress, anxiety and depression. Children pull because it feels good or fills some kind of need, but hardly ever because they want to become ugly or to purposely disfigure themselves.

Trichotillomania is believed to affect 2-5% of the population (you see, your child is not alone, or really that strange at all!) and 80-90% of reported cases are women, although in children the percentage is closer to a 50-50% ratio of girls to boys. The average age of onset is 11, however pulling can start at any age. Some children may stop on their own. However, many do not, and we encourage parents to understand the condition fully and to get involved in finding a treatment as soon as possible. The earlier neural patterns that develop during habits are altered, the easier it will be for your child to be cured.

Common feelings

As a parent you will go through a variety of emotions, and just the ups and downs can be very wearing on parents and children alike. You will feel frustration and despair, followed by elation when they start to improve, only to be disappointed when your child starts pulling again. You will probably not understand what is going on and not really believe that your child cannot control his or her behavior. You will most likely feel embarrassed by your child's appearance, sometimes to the extent of not wanting to talk about it, even with health care professionals. You will probably also feel guilt, as if there is something that you could have done differently that would change the situation. You may also feel overwhelmed and confused by all of the conflicting advice and thoughts. While all of these feelings are perfectly natural reactions, you must understand the condition fully in order to dispel these emotions and replace them with more constructive and positive feelings of hope, encouragement and positivism.

Belief is key in treatment of habits and OCD conditions. There have been many studies around why groups such as Alcoholics Anonymous are effective, and there is very strong evidence that an important factor is seeing others who have achieved a goal. Being in a group that cultivates positivism and a 'can do' attitude has a huge impact on eventual success. Therefore it is important to both stay positive for your child, as well as to surround the child with positive support groups and role models.

Just remember, your child will also be going through his own set of (often very similar) emotions, such as shame, guilt and not being able to understand why he cannot stop.

In this case you need to be a strong support for your child to be able to work through his emotions with you, without judgment or your own baggage interfering. In order to do this you must understand the condition and have complete compassion for the sufferer. Have you ever tried to stop smoking, chew on your fingernails or follow a diet? If so then you know that often these things are much more difficult than they look. With this in mind, put yourself in your child's shoes and exhibit compassion at all times when dealing with your child.

Compassion is key.

Your child will pick up on your own attitude and outlook. A

sense of confidence and belief in your child, coupled with

compassion and understanding will make recovery not only

possible, but a less stressful and isolating time for all concerned.

Your attitude and outlook means everything, and your child will follow your lead.

Working with Your Child

No matter what the age of your child, your approach should be similar. Your goal is to establish trust in each other, to show your confidence in your child and to boost their self-esteem when they are feeling low.

Explaining what Trichotillomania is, how many people of all sorts are affected, showing him the websites, resources and stories of others and thus showing him that he is not a freak is an important first step.

Explaining to your son or daughter that you understand what they are going through and that you know that they can't 'just stop' will be a relief to your child who surely feels that no one understands him. You will become a safe haven for your child who will come to you more and more often for help. Show your child that you are there to help them put a structured plan in place and that this will be a gradual, but positive process. Often verbalizing your own experience of difficulties in changing your behavior (whether it be dieting, nail biting, smoking, etc) can show your child better than through words that you understand his situation and that he truly is not alone.

Do not set time limits or ultimatums, or use rewards. These will only put pressure on your child and often result in more lost confidence when they cannot reach the goals that have been set.

Above all, never chastise, ridicule or punish your child in hopes that you can control their condition. This will not work and will only backfire, making them more secretive and more ashamed, exacerbating the problem.

All of your actions should be based on building confidence and trust in your child. When in doubt, ask yourself if the message you are sending is a constructive, collaborative and positive one that will set your child up for success.

Your Philosophy as a Parent

This is a good time to reevaluate your philosophy as a parent. Do you even have one? To be an effective parent, it is good to have a well thought out philosophy of how you want to parent; a philosophy that is in line with your beliefs and goals for your child and family. A philosophy will give very important coherence to your parenting, but will also help you in those frustrating moments when you aren't sure how to react. In these moments you can always fall back on your beliefs and ask yourself what actions would be in line with that philosophy. In the raising of my children, I have found that the philosophy that their father and I established at the very beginning of their babyhood has helped us throughout their childhood.

Your philosophy as a parent, and how you treat your children about other subjects will have an impact on your ability to deal with your child's' Trichotillomania. A good way to develop your philosophy is to read books (see our list of recommended resources), talk to parents that you admire and discuss with your parenting partner your goals, and wishes for your children and your parenting.

Think about what values you want to instill and how to exhibit these to your children (children do as you do and not as you say), how you want to discipline, what kind of relationship you see with them in the long run, etc.

For hair pulling treatments, a philosophy of caring support, encouraging confidence and belief and a strong structure for the child to function in is the most effective.

Treatment and support

Just as there are many different sufferers of trich, there are many different types of treatments, from medication to self-awareness training. There is no known 'cure' for Trichotillomania but there are treatment options available. Discovering ways to control hair-pulling impulses can help a patient become pull free. Cognitive behavior therapy, stress-control medications, and hair pulling support groups have all proven as an effective way to control symptoms. Cognitive Behavior Therapy trains patients in self-monitoring, identifying and responding to high-risk solutions, assessing the function of the pull, confronting realizations, and developing mindfulness.

I suggest working with a mix of methods in order to find the one or combination that is most effective for your child's particular case. Most importantly, it is important for those who suffer from

Trich to know that although it can be difficult to stop hair pulling, **it is possible!**

You will find many different methods in the Trich Stop Manual and Workbook, and we suggest you try all of them with your child. Often a combination of treatments will prove to be the most effective.

Therapy or no?

While we encourage suffers to give therapy a go (after all, we use accountants and lawyers for specialized help, why not a therapist), many children (and parents for that matter) balk at therapy. It seems to concretize the abnormality and shame. We suggest starting with the Trich Stop home program to give the sufferer some confidence and structure in the privacy of their own home. Once they are feeling good with the advances they are making, you can try a therapist and see if this is right for your child. Above all do not force your child to see a therapist or do anything in their treatment that they do not want to do. A child's acceptance is often gradual, and respecting their own rhythm sends the important message that you have confidence in them and will allow them to have at least some control in their own life.

Setbacks and how to deal with them

One last word on setbacks: setbacks are a normal part of the process and you should be prepared, and prepare for your child for them. Aim for gradual healing rather than a radical cold turkey approach, which will only cause frustration and loss of confidence. Retraining the neural patterns as well as putting healing systems in place take time, so allow your family the time to heal together. When your child has a setback, don't make a big deal out of it. Just pick yourselves back up, dust yourselves off, explain the gradual nature of recovery to your child and start again. Explain to your child that having been able to make any progress at all shows that it is possible. Now it just needs to become ingrained behavior, which it will, with enough time and practice.

Most of all teach your child to be kind to himself.

Top Tips

- o Show your confidence in your child as a person

- o Compassion and belief are ESSENTIAL

- o Encourage your child to use the Trich Stop Journal and Trich Stop Oil

- o Modifying the pulling behavior to stroking (using some sort of all natural oil) is essential to develop new neural pathways and instill long lasting results

- o Encourage your child to try many different methods to find the ones that work best for him or her

- o Never chastise, punish, ridicule or force your child in any way

Recommended resources

A Good Enough Parent - Bruno Bettleheim

The Power of Habit - Charles Duhigg

The Perfect Pull – Lindsay Woolman

The Dragon Who Pulled Her Scales – Michael Davidson

www.trich.org

www.trichotillomania.co.uk

How to Use the Trich Stop System With Your Child

The Trich Stop System has been designed to include many different methods. It has been created in a way so that the trich sufferer can develop their own personalized treatment. You should work with your child to help him do just that with the aid of the manual and workbook.

You will need to follow your child's lead when helping them work through their condition, including with the Trich Stop System. Allow them to 'own' the manual. Encourage them to use it as they would like – writing in it, doodling, whatever helps them express themselves.

Don't ask to see their journal or any private writings and don't look at them unless they ask you to. Don't even 'check up' to see if they have been writing in their journal. This is a moment to establish trust and confidence, which will, in turn, help them discover confidence in themselves.

Encourage them to keep some kind of oil (we recommend the Trich Stop Oil) to discreetly use then they are having urges. It is important to help them begin the reflex of stroking rather than pulling (see behavior modification in the Trich Stop Manual).

Remember - this is their journey and you are there only as support.

If you liked this...

We hope you find this guide helpful and full of great ideas. If you would like to know more about how you can continue to fight against Trichotillomania, then visit us on www.Trichotillomaniastop.com.

A Special Offer

As one of our Trich Stop community we'd like to extend to you two special offers:

- a 10% discount on our Trich Stop Vitamin Supplement that gives you all the dietary needs and proven amino acids to beat Trich urges and start growing back luxurious and healthy hair quickly.

- a 10% discount on a refill of the Trich Stop Oil

If you are interested just contact me at amy@foxwellassociates.com, mentioning 'special offer' in the subject.

We'd Love to Hear from You

We believe that a community is a powerful thing. If you have any thoughts, comments, feedback or suggestions then please feel free to send them through to us at comments@foxwellassociates.com. If there is anything you have done that you think would be beneficial to other Trich sufferers and their parents, or unique ways you have used the ideas presented here, then send them in. Here at Trich Stop, we are always happy to work as a team.

Notes

Welcome to the Trich Stop Kit

Congratulations. By reading this you are taking the first step to a new you. I am delighted to share this method that helped me to stop pulling my hair out and is sure to give you immediate results. I have spent much time researching and developing this kit for it to be as effective as possible. All you need to do to see lasting results is to follow the instructions and most of all, be kind to yourself as you embark on this journey.

My best,

Amy Foxwell

A Word about the Trich Stop System

Whether you have been battling with Trichotillomania for several years, or have just begun to see symptoms of this condition, you must personally resolve to take control of the situation. And that is what the Trich Stop System is for; to help you succeed in tackling your own personal Trichotillomania condition. Everyone is different and everyone's condition is different. However there are some underlying causes and remedies that are common to everyone. You will need to understand as much as you can about your condition and then put these action steps in place to help you beat it. The key to know is that this can be done. YOU CAN STOP PULLING YOUR HAIR OUT. You just need the support and plan in place to help you. And that is where the Trich Stop System comes in. Read this manual and begin the steps, using the Trich Stop Hairgrowth Oil (see page 32 for more information or refer to: http://trichotillomaniastop.com/hair-growth-oil/) to help you achieve your goals. You will see immediate improvements. Congratulate yourself and recognize that if you can make these first steps towards improvement, then the final goal of stopping your hair pulling is within your reach.

So, now that you know that you will succeed, let's get started.

Background

What is Hair Pulling Disorder, or Trichotillomania?

Trichotillomania is classified as an impulse control disorder. People who suffer from this hair pulling disorder have the uncontrollable urge to pull out hair from their scalp or other parts of their body. Patients are unable to stop this behavior, even as their hair becomes thinner and results in noticeable bald patches. It is more than just a nervous habit, which can be controlled through simply by deciding to stop. This repetitive behavior is often self-destructive and distressing to the sufferer.

Hair pulling is not limited to the scalp. Patients tend to pluck other hairy areas, such as eyelashes, eyebrows, or body hair. Most often patients pull hairs one-by-one, often targeting hair of a specific color or texture. Similar body focused-repetitive behaviors include skin picking, lip biting and nail biting. Despite the desire to quit harming their bodies in such a way, people who suffer from Trich have a hard time controlling these urges. This not only results in physical impairments but also significant emotional distress. It is by no means a patient's fault for being unable to control such behavior.

What Causes Trichotillomania?

Research of causes and treatments of Trichotillomania are still in the early stages. Studies have shown evidence that indicates Trich to be a neurobiological disorder and may be linked to one's genetic makeup. Hair pulling is often triggered by stress, anxiety and depression. People with Trichotillomania generally have a neurologically based, often genetic predisposition to pull their hair as a self-soothing mechanism. 80% of hair pullers also report an itch-like urge to pull and there may well be a cause similar to folliculitis (inflammation of the hair root) or an irritation to the very natural and normal skin yeast, Malassezia.

Patients have a hard time controlling this obsessive compulsive behavior due to the vicious cycle of complications that stems from Trich. Hair pulling worsens the emotional instability that causes a patient to pull. Pulling momentarily satisfies patients but in the long run results in serious emotional consequences, such as severe self-consciousness, poor self-image, low self-esteem, and other lifestyle setbacks. Individuals who pull tend to feel "freakish" or "crazy" because of the abnormal behavior and its effects.

Who Suffers from Trichotillomania?

Trichotillomania is believed to affect 2-5% of the population and 80-90% of reported cases are women. The average age of onset is 11, however pulling can start at any age. Children under the age of 6 years old usually stop hair pulling after 12 months. The diagnosis criteria for Trich in the mental health field include a presence of multiple symptoms:

1. Hair pulling that results in noticeable hair loss

2. Relief and gratification during pulling

3. Increased tension when resisting pulling

4. Significant impairment in social functions due to pulling

The Phases of Trichotillomania

There are three main phases to Trichotillomania:

1. An initial experience of tension accompanied by a desire to pull out some hair.

2. Hair pulling begins and feels good, with a sense of relief, as well as some excitement.

3. Once the hair is pulled, the sufferer feels guilt, remorse, and shame. Attempts are made to cover the bald patches with scarves, hats, wigs, eyeliner and sufferers begin hiding at this point, or to feel intensely humiliated.

Treatment and Support

There is no known 'cure' for Trichotillomania but there are treatment options available. Discovering ways to control hair-pulling impulses can help a patient become pull free. Cognitive behavior therapy, stress-control medications, and hair pulling support groups have all proven as an effective way to control symptoms. Cognitive Behavior Therapy trains patients in self-monitoring, identifying and responding to high-risk solutions,

assessing the function of the pull, confronting realizations, and

developing mindfulness.

It is important for those who suffer from Trich to know that

although it can be difficult to stop hair pulling, it is possible!

Trich Stop Tools

The Success Mindset: Using Visualization

The indispensible first step to getting the things that you want out of life is this: decide what you want. - Ben Stein

Visualisation is a powerful tool that many successful athletes, businessmen and leaders use on a regular basis. It consists of picturing exactly what you want in order to help you get it. The practice has been the object of many studies and is based on the fact that your brain cannot recognise the difference between reality and imagination. So that if you imagine something often and clearly enough the brain will take it as truth and will do everything in its power to treat these visualisations as reality and help you achieve them.

Some guidelines for visualisation:

- Be very clear with exactly what your vision is. See it in as much detail as possible. Include sounds, smells, and your emotions, with as much detail to make it real for your brain as possible. Imagine how you feel as you go out without any make up on, as someone compliments you on your beautiful eyes. Remember – you are programming your brain to achieve whatever you are picturing, so make it good.

- Visualise in an active, present tense. 'I am proud hearing a person compliment me on y beautiful hair.' rather than 'I would be happy if…, or 'I am happy that I have beautiful luxurious hair.', rather than 'When I don't have any more bald spots I will be happy…'.

- When a negative thought comes in to quash your vision isolate the thought, turn it into black and white, cut the sound off, reduce it to a speck and then imagine blowing the negative thought away.

- Visualise on a daily basis. When you get up in the morning and before you go to sleep. Consider putting together a vision board, full of images and quotes that will inspire you when you contemplate it.

- Include every detail in your life, not just your hair pulling goals. Imagine the activities that you excel at, the time you spend with your friends, a full life like you want to live it.

- Remember - the sky is the limit. The more you wish for, the more you will get. If you can't even imagine success, then it is sure that it will elude you.

- Fill out a chart like this to get started. Be sure each goal is measurable, detailed and has a time limit.

Relations	Activities	School	Hair Pulling	Personal

Time and again visualization has been proven a valuable free resource, so tap into it.

Auto-hypnosis

Using auto-hypnosis can help you conquer that part of you that is working against your own best interest and harness the power of your own mind to beat Trichotillomania. Consciously, you may know all the good reasons not to pull, but you need to feel, not just think, differently about pulling your hair out. The basic thing to know about auto-hypnosos is that the mind is most receptive when it is calm and the body is relaxed. So the key to success in auto-hypnosis is simply relaxing the body and quieting the mind.

Follow this 10-step process to use auto-hypnosis as a part of your Trich cure:

1. Develop the suggestion that you will use during your auto-hypnosos. It must be:

   o   positive, with no negative words.

- short, between 6 and 15 words.

- meaningful, this is what you really want to happen.

- possible, something you can achieve. Avoid absolutes and time limits.

- focused, tackle one suggestion at a time, not many different wishes.

- For example "Every day I do not pull out any eyelashes."

2. Write your suggestion on a piece of paper

- in clear, neat handwriting.

- write as if you were writing to your best friend or lover.

- concentrate and write slowly thinking about the meaning of the words as you write each of them.

- Repeat the message to yourself, preferably out loud, listening carefully to yourself, and to your words. Think clearly about their meaning.

3. Find a place where you can relax and be by yourself. You might put on some of your favorite music in the background (no

singing).

4. You should carry out the auto-hypnosis programming three
   times a day:

   o When you wake up in the morning - as soon as possible
      after awakening.

   o In the middle of the day, best just after lunch.

   o Just before going to sleep at night

5. Sit or lie comfortably and find something to look at and focus
   on. Take three deep breaths, letting yourself relax all over
   and feeling the stress and tension leaving your body with
   each exhalation. Breath in serenity, breath out tension.

6. Close your eyes and hold the last breath for at least 10 seconds
   then slowly let it all out, letting all the tension in all of your
   muscles flow outward with that last exhalation.

7. Now that you are relaxed, and breathing evenly and smoothly,

begin to count backwards from 5 to 1. As you count you feel yourself relaxing deeper and deeper with each and every breath you take, with every number you count.

8. When you reach the count of 1, feel yourself drop quickly and deeply into a very comfortable and relaxed state of mind.

9. Now begin to say, in your mind, not out loud, the words you wish to program into your subconscious, repeating the phrase 20 times. To help you keep count, each time you say the phrase, move the tip of a finger to the tip of your thumb. Do not hurry. Go slow and deep. After you have mastered the process, it becomes automatic and you don't have to pay too much attention to either the hand movements or the words themselves. This might take a few days.

10. As you improve, begin to focus on relaxing deeper and deeper, drifting away, just letting yourself completely relax. Don't rush the process. When you find yourself able to think of other things, begin to parallel the suggestion with the

following thoughts:

- "Each and every word you hear me say takes you deeper and deeper into a very beneficial state of relaxation."

- "You can hear my words giving you suggestions, these suggestions will make your life better and happier."

- "Each and every time I do this exercise the effect is stronger and more beneficial. The suggestion is helping improve my life more and more as I move deeper and deeper during the exercises."

8 Step Trich Stop System

This 8 step system is a proven system for helping you to stop hair puling, no matter how long you have been pulling. These 7 steps, along with the tools above will help you put in place an effective plan for your successful Trich cure.

1. Before you begin

Be kind to yourself. You are not alone and you are not a freak. Trich is a legitimate condition that you suffer from. You can beat it, but it is hard, so be kind with yourself as you move through the system. If you slip and do pull don't berate yourself, just accept that it is a part of the cure and get back on the plan. I often compared myself to my husband who was quitting smoking, and tried to be as kind and understanding to myself as I was with him. It's TOUGH, but YOU CAN DO IT.

2. Recognize The Condition

Acknowledge that you have a problem. The first thing to realize is that you suffer from treatable disorder, not something due to willpower or lack thereof. The disorder arises as a result of genetic makeup, moods, and your background and is a condition in need of treating, not something to beat yourself up over. On the other hand, don't convince yourself that nothing is wrong. Trichotillomania can be considered a form of self-harm, and like all forms of self-harm, Trichotillomania can become an addictive behavior, so you need to recognize and treat it as such. My big breakthrough was when I finally realized that my Trich was a legitimate condition. This freed me of guilt and shame and allowed me to move forward to looking for the treatment that best suited me and my own personal version of the condition.

3. Identify When You Pull

Know your triggers. Hair pulling becomes addictive because of the natural pain-killing 'buzz' that self-harm gives us; the body's natural morphine kicks in. When do you pull your hair out? In the evening when watching television? When speaking to an annoying friend on the phone? When reading or working on the computer? Make a list of your triggers and next to each write down an alternative activity that would make you feel better in these contexts.

The initial cause of trichotillomania could be genetic and/or environmental, and researchers see similarities with the triggers for obsessive-compulsive disorder. Distressing experiences or disturbed relationships with family might be behind the development of this disorder, and one study has shown that over two-thirds of sufferers have experienced at least one traumatic event in their lives, with a fifth of them diagnosed with post-traumatic stress disorder. This has led researchers to believe that it may be a way to cope for some sufferers. Therefore in your own case, regardless of what may or may not have brought on the condition, consider what kinds of situations cause you to resort to hair pulling. Do you only do it when you're depressed? Angry? Confused? Frustrated? Bored? Once you identify and understand what triggers your hair pulling, you can find other, more positive ways of coping.

4. Write Down When You Pull and Keep a Journal

Keep a journal or a chart of your hair-pulling episodes. Through writing you can get a good idea of the times, the triggers, and the impact of your hair pulling. Record the date, time, location, and number of hairs you pull and what you used to pull them. Write down your thoughts or feelings when you pull as well. This is a good way of relieving yourself of the guilt and shame, and of expressing how the hair pulling is impacting your life in general. You will begin to identify your weak moments and mental states. By being more aware of these moments and feelings you will begin to master them. You may be surprised to see how much hair you have pulled or how much time you have spent doing so. You may also be surprised to find times that you pull that you were not aware of, or feelings that reoccur. You will also want to use a journal to express your emotions. Write out a list of the consequences you've experienced as a result of the hair pulling. It might include comments from people you have endured, having to go to great lengths with eyeliner or head coverings. It should also include the relationship consequences, such as not going on a date or to spending time with people because you're afraid they will find out about your hair pulling.

5. Make a Plan

Develop a 'Recognize, Interrupt, and Alternatives Plan' to help you stop pulling your hair. This consists of noticing when you feel like pulling your hair and then interrupting the feelings and urges by listening to visualization and positive reminders in your head. Then, choose an alternative action, something that will relax you or deal with the feelings that bring on the compulsion to pull. Alternative ways of expressing your emotions and might be deep breathing and clearing your mind, rehearsing your visualization, drawing or writing, calling a friend that knows about your condition or not, beginning a manual activity such as beading, needlepoint or video games. Many people have found using physical reminders effective, such as wearing weights that pull on the arms, gloves or fake fingernails as a reminder and a hindrance to pulling.

6. Keep Your Trich Stop Oil Close at Hand

The Trich Stop Hairgrowth Oil (for more information:

http://trichotillomaniastop.com/hair-growth-oil/) was the

absolute key to my success to stop pulling my eyelashes and hair

out. It has been specially developed to calm and sooth your

follicles as well as stimulate re-growth. I developed it as an aid

to help me with my own condition and would use it whenever I

had an urge to pull as an alternative action. I suffered from itchy,

irritated follicles and the oil was a relief for the 'physical' and

uncomfortable sensation pushing me to pull. In addition the

oiliness made it difficult to pull and it was a comfort that I was

nourishing the hair follicles and encouraging re-growth. Keep

your serum with you at times that you are susceptible to pull and

choose it as an alternative action as well as a soother and a

reminder that you are experiencing your triggers and that you

can overcome them. (see page 32 for a special reader offer).

7. Find What Works For You

Every Trich suffer is different. Use the Trich Stop System to put a personalized plan in place for your own hair pulling condition. You will want to experiment with different steps of the process to identify what is the most effective for you.

8. Use Auxiliary Activities

Do not skip using the auxiliary activities such as visualization and auto-hypnosis. They are powerful tools and in conjunction with the Trich Stop System will be sure to lead you to beating Trich successfully!

Trich Stop Top Tips

These tips will help you beat Trich today!

Systems and structures are the key

Do not leave your treatment to chance. Put in place concrete structures and a plan to eliminate the chaos and give you guidelines and a context as support. This is key to success.

If you slip up

Do not beat yourself up over any slip-ups. This will happen and is a natural part of the process. Just use the mistake as a learning experience to better understand your Trich and continue to develop the best solution for your personal version of the condition. Write down your mistakes in your journal and suggest to yourself possible solutions. The goal will be not to go cold turkey which could cause unbearable frustration that will lead to certain relapse, but to gradually pull less and less in a structured way, with pulling episodes becoming less frequent so that one day you wake up and you haven't pulled for a very long time!

Use distraction

Get into the habit of doing something else when you get the urge to pull hair out, such as going for a walk, doing needlepoint, writing in your journal, etc. Distraction isn't just about doing something else, it's about retraining the brain to the point where it starts to feel more natural not to pull in response to your trigger times.

Successfully identify trigger times

Of course, sometimes you will find yourself pulling at your hair without even having been aware of any triggers (although there is always one). So you might want to use something to physically help identify your triggers such as weights on your arms during danger times when you might become in a trancelike state and not realize your pulling activity (such as reading or watching television).

Forget the mirror

Stop looking in the mirror! Examining the area will only focus your attention on it and your failure to control yourself. This means even after you have pulled to see the damage. Just ignore the area and the next thing you know, when you do catch a glimpse of yourself, SURPRISE, you'll have new hair where it used to be bald. It seems like such a simple thing to do, but stopping myself from looking in the mirror constantly was one of the major keys to my peace of mind and success.

Watch your diet

Having a healthy body is key to laying the foundations to successfully beat Trich and grow your hair back. There are many studies that show that nutrition can contribute to exacerbating urges to pull. Cut out processed and junk foods, eat a balanced healthy diet and exercise when you can. Exercise improves circulation throughout your body, including your scalp, which can result in faster hair growth and soothed follicles. Eat the foods that your body needs to beat Trich, keep hair follicles healthy and grow strong hair back quickly:

· Vitamin A is essential for hair growth. Natural food sources include mango, orange, carrot, sweet potato, and squash. But don't take supplements as too much can actually cause hair loss.

· Vitamin B boosts the production of hemoglobin, which helps follicles receive enough oxygen to stay healthy and promote hair growth. Eat potatoes, garbanzo beans/chickpeas, chicken breast, oatmeal, pork loin, and roast beef.

· Potassium. The highest concentrations are found in bananas and the added potassium helps to balance out deficiencies that can contribute to hair pulling urges.

· Folic acid is found in collard greens, lentils, garbanzo beans/chickpeas, papaya, peas, and asparagus, folic acid contributes to natural hair regrowth.

· Vitamin E also helps blood circulate to the scalp and improve hair growth and can be found in most cereals, almonds, safflower oil, corn oil, and soybean oil.

· Vitamin C is required for the development of collagen, which is necessary for growing strong hair. Eat kiwi fruit, guava, red peppers, and oranges.

I also have a Trich Stop Vitamin Supplement that has been specially developed for Trich sufferers. I have found it very effective in curbing the urge to pull as well as growing back hair.

Contact me at amy@foxwellassociates.com for more information.

2. Go online, use forums and get help!

Use the online (and offline) support groups that are available. However be judicious when choosing the one you will participate in. Try out several and give them a chance until you find the one that matches your personal style. Be careful to choose a support group that is positive, believes in a cure and is looking to help you in your success, not one that is full of complainers and moaners and people that just want to commiserate together. Those kind of groups will surely fail as they have already decided to fail in their minds. Remember Trich is a condition and so you need the right mental state to beat it. A positive outlook is key, so surround yourself with positive people. Choose a support group that has people that have successfully beat Trich – by surrounding yourself with winners you too will become a winner.

Consider starting therapy and getting professional help. While I beat Trich without it, I see no shame in getting professional help. Why reinvent the wheel after all? Get a therapist and take advantage of the wisdom and experience that has gone before you, as well as benefit from the contacts and resources that will become available to you. People use an accountant, lawyer, doctor or other professional that is trained in their area for your other needs, so why not do the same for this very real condition that has such a big impact on your life?

Facts About Hair Growth

Human hair naturally falls out and therefore your hair WILL grow back, even after being repeatedly pulled out. Here are some facts to about hair growth:

- Human hair grows approximately 1/4 to 1/2 inch per month, or 6 inches per year.

- Heat, as well as Vitamin D from the sun can stimulate growth, so getting sun on your hair will make your hair may grow back faster.

- Your body is constantly shedding hair. Hair follicles go through three phases during their life cycle: the anagen phase for about three years, a transitional phase and the telogen phase for about three months, when hair rests. Once this phase ends, the hair is shed.

o   The scalp sheds about 100 hairs per day. Because each strand is in a different phase, normal hair loss is unnoticeable. At any given period, you have approximately 100,000 hairs on your head.

o   Eyelashes naturally grow, fall out, and grow back again. Eyelashes also go through the 3 phases of hair: growth, transition, and resting phases. The 1st phase is when eyelashes grow and lasts up to a maximum of 45 days. After which, they go through the 2nd phase which may last up to 3 weeks, when the eyelashes stop growing. In the 3rd phase, the lashes are not growing and stay for approximately 100 days before they then fall out.

o   It normally takes up to 8 weeks for an eyelash to grow back fully.

Using the Trich Stop System Worksheet and Journal

Use the following three steps along with the Trich Stop Manual and Trich Stop Serum to put a structure and plan in place to beat your condition.

1. Recognize The Condition

Acknowledge that you have a problem. The first thing to realize is that you suffer from treatable disorder, not something due to willpower or lack thereof. The disorder arises as a result of genetic makeup, moods, and your background and is a condition in need of treating, not something to beat yourself up over.

2. Identify When You Pull

Know your triggers. When do you pull your hair out? In the evening when watching tv or reading? When speaking to your ex-boyfriend on the phone? When working on your homework? Make a list of your triggers and next to each write down an alternative activity that would make you feel better in these contexts.

3. Write Down When You Pull and Keep a Journal

Keep a journal or a chart of your hair-pulling episodes. Through writing you can get a good idea of the times, the triggers, and the impact of your hair pulling. This is a good way of relieving yourself of the guilt and shame, and of expressing how the hair pulling is impacting your life in general. You will begin to identify your weak moments and mental states. By being more aware of these moments and feelings you will begin to master them. You will also want to use a journal to express your emotions. Write out a list of the consequences you've experienced as a result of the hair pulling.

4. How to fill out the worksheet and journal

Keep a regular journal, filling it out daily with your Trich related experiences. We have included the first few pages to get you started.

Comments and observations from others:

Include comments you have endured and any observations friends, family or strangers have made about your appearance or condition, and how you felt.

Behavioral consequences to my pulling

Include any behavior that is a consequence of your condition (having to go to great lengths with eyeliner or head coverings, etc.), and how you felt.

Relationship consequences to my pulling

Include the relationship consequences, such as not going on a date or to spending time with people because you're afraid they will find out about your hair pulling, and how you felt.

Triggers

Make a list of your triggers and next to each write down an alternative activity that would make you feel better in these contexts.

Tracking Chart

Fill out a chart like the one on the next page to track your pulling

behavior and emotions:

Date, time	Place	Trigger	How many hairs pulled	What used was to pull?	Thoughts	Feelings	Possible other activities

My Trich Stop Success Journal

Comments and observations from others

Comments:

_____

_____

_____

My feelings:

_____

_____

_____

Comments:

_____

_____

_____

My feelings:

_____

_____

_____

Comments:

_____

_____

_____

My feelings:

_____

_____

_____

Behavioral consequences to my pulling

Behavior:

_____

_____

_____

My feelings:

_____

_____

_____

Behavior:

_____

_____

_____

My feelings:

_____

_____

_____

Behavior:

_____

_____

_____

My feelings:

_____

_____

_____

Relationship consequences to my pulling

Behavior:

_____

_____

_____

My feelings:

_____

_____

_____

Behavior:

_____

_____

_____

My feelings:

_____

_____

_____

Behavior:

_____

_____

_____

My feelings:

_____

_____

_____

Triggers

Trigger:

_____

_____

_____

Alternative activity:

_____

_____

_____

Trigger:

_____

_____

_____

Alternative activity:

_____

_____

_____

Trigger:

_____

_____

_____

Alternative activity:

_____

_____

_____

Tracking Chart

Date, time	Place	Trigger	How many hairs pulled	What used was to pull?	Thoughts	Feelings	Possible other activities

Notes